KIDNEY HEALTH DIET PLAN COOK BOOK

The Perfect Kidney Health Diet: Recipes for Vitality and Wellness

REX LEWIS

Table of Contents

Introduction

Comprehending Kidney Health Is Essential For Sustaining General Well-Being, As The Kidneys Are Necessary For Filtering And Eliminating Waste Products From The Blood, Controlling Fluid Balance, And Managing Electrolyte Levels In The Body. **Here Are Some Crucial Factors To Consider Regarding Kidney Health:**

1. Structure and Purpose:

• The Kidneys Are Kidney-Shaped Organs Situated Bilaterally Beside The Spine, Beneath The Ribcage.

• The Kidneys Filter Blood By Eliminating Waste Products, Excess

Fluids, And Electrolytes, Which Are Expelled As Urine.

• The Kidneys Are Involved In Maintaining Blood Pressure And Producing Hormones That Stimulate The Creation Of Red Blood Cells.

2. Typical Kidney Disorders:

• Chronic Kidney Disease (CKD) Is A Persistent Illness Characterized By The Steady Decline In Kidney Function Over An Extended Period. Causes Comprise Diabetes, Hypertension, And Other Fundamental Health Disorders.

• Kidney Stones Are Solid Deposits That Develop In The Kidneys And Can Lead To Pain And Obstruction In The Urinary Canal.

Urinary Tract Infections (Utis) Are Infections That Impact The Urinary System, Which Includes The Kidneys.

3. Factors That Increase the Likelihood of a Negative Outcome:

• **Diabetes:** Poorly Managed Diabetes Can Lead To Kidney Damage In The Long Term.

• Hypertension, Or High Blood Pressure, Can Put A Burden On The Kidneys And Cause Harm.

• Family History Can Indicate A Hereditary Propensity To Kidney Issues If Close Relatives Have Been Affected.

Age Is A Factor That Raises The Likelihood Of Renal Issues.

4. Kidney Health Maintenance:

• Stay Hydrated By Drinking An Adequate Amount Of Water To Eliminate Toxins And Reduce The Risk Of Kidney Stones.

• A Balanced Diet With Fruits, Vegetables, Whole Grains, And Lean Proteins Promotes Kidney Function.

• Limit Salt Consumption To Prevent High Blood Pressure And Maintain Optimal Renal Function.

Regular Exercise Assists In Maintaining A Healthy Weight And Blood Pressure.

5. Monitoring Renal Function:

• Regular Check-Ups, Including Periodic Blood Pressure Checks And Renal Function Testing, Can Help Identify Concerns At An Early Stage.

• Blood And Urine Tests Can Evaluate Kidney Function By Measuring Creatinine, Blood Urea Nitrogen (Bun), And Other Indicators.

6. Requesting Medical Consultation:

• If You Have Chronic Symptoms Such As Changes In Urine Color, Frequency, Or Pain, Seek Advice From A Healthcare Expert.

Manage Medical Diseases Such As Diabetes And Hypertension With The Assistance Of A Healthcare Expert.

It Is Crucial To Comprehend And Take Proactive Measures To Preserve Renal Health In Order To Prevent Kidney Disorders And Promote Overall Well-Being. For Tailored Advice And Support, It Is Crucial To Seek The Expertise Of A Healthcare Professional If You Have Particular Concerns Or Conditions.

CHAPTER ONE
Principles of Renal Function

The Kidneys Are Essential Organs That Perform Multiple Processes Crucial For The Body's Well-Being. Here Are The Fundamental Aspects Of Kidney Function:

1. Blood Filtration: The Main Role Of The Kidneys Is To Filter The Blood, Eliminating Waste Products And Excess Chemicals.

• Blood Containing Waste Materials Including Urea, Creatinine, And Excess Salts Reaches The Kidneys Via The Renal Arteries.

2. Urine Production: The Strained Blood Flows Via Minuscule Units In The Kidneys Known As Nephrons.

• Nephrons Selectively Reabsorb Vital Chemicals Such As Water, Glucose, And Electrolytes Into The Bloodstream.

Remaining Trash And Surplus Substances Combine To Create Urine.

3. Fluid and Electrolyte Balance Regulation:

• The Kidneys Assist In Regulating The Equilibrium Of Fluids And Electrolytes (Sodium, Potassium, Chloride) In The Body.

Proper Electrolyte Balance Is Essential For Neuron Function, Muscular Contraction, And Cellular Activity.

4. Acid-Base Balance:

• The Kidneys Manage The Body's Acid-Base Balance By Excreting Hydrogen Ions And Reabsorbing Bicarbonate Ions, Which Helps To Keep The Blood Ph Steady.

5. Regulation of Blood Pressure:

• The Renal Renin-Angiotensin-Aldosterone System Is Crucial For Blood Pressure Regulation.

• The Kidneys Secrete Renin When Blood Pressure Is Low, Triggering A Sequence Of Actions To Boost Blood Volume And Elevate Blood Pressure.

6. Regulation of Erythropoiesis:

• The Kidneys Secrete Erythropoietin, A Hormone That Promotes The Generation Of Red Blood Cells In The Bone Marrow When Oxygen Levels In The Blood Are Low.

7. Detoxification:

• The Kidneys Aid In The Removal Of Different Metabolic Waste Products, Medications, And Poisons From The Body.

8. Vitamin D Activation:

• The Kidneys Activate Vitamin D, Crucial For Absorbing Calcium And Phosphate In The Intestines To Support Bone Health.

The Kidneys Are Essential For Maintaining Internal Equilibrium In The Body Through Blood Filtration, Fluid And Electrolyte Regulation, Blood Pressure Control, Hormone Production, And Waste Elimination. Any Decline In Kidney Function Can Result In A Range Of Health Issues, Highlighting The Significance Of Preserving Kidney Health Through A Balanced Lifestyle And Routine Medical Examinations.

Kidney Problem Symptoms

Renal Issues Can Present In Diverse Ways, With Signs And Symptoms Differing Based On The Particular Illness. Below Are Typical Indicators

That Could Suggest Possible Renal Issues:

1. Urination Alterations:

• **Frequent Urination**: Experiencing A Higher Frequency Of Urination Than Normal.

• **Urgency:** Abrupt, Intense Need To Urinate.

• Difficulty Or Discomfort During Urination: Discomfort Or Discomfort Experienced During Urinating.

2. Alterations in Urine Color: Blood in Pee (Hematuria): Pink, Crimson, or Brown Urine May Suggest The Presence Of Blood.

Foamy Or Bubbly Pee May Indicate The Presence Of Protein In The Urine.

3. Edema: Swelling

• Edema Is The Accumulation Of Fluid Causing Swelling In The Hands, Feet, Face, Or Other Parts Of The Body.

4. Fatigue and Weakness:

• Prolonged Exhaustion And Debility, Maybe Due To Anemia Or The Accumulation Of Toxins In The Body.

5. Back Pain Or Flank Pain:

• Pain In The Lower Back Or Sides (Flanks), Where The Kidneys Are Placed.

6. Hypertension: Hypertension Can both Result From And Lead To Renal Issues.

7. Appetite Alterations: Loss Of Appetite Or Sudden Weight Loss Without Explanation.

8. Electrolyte Imbalance: Symptoms Like Muscle Cramps, Weakness, Or Irregular Heart Rhythms Might Arise From Electrolyte Imbalances Caused By Kidney Disease.

9. Nauseated and Vomiting: Feeling Nauseated And Vomiting May Be Linked To The Accumulation Of Waste Materials In The Bloodstream.

10. Pruritus and Dermatological Eruption: Accumulation Of Waste Materials In The Blood Can Result In Skin Problems, Leading To Itching And Rashes.

11. Dyspnea: Fluid Retention And Anemia Related To Kidney Issues Can Result In Respiratory Difficulties.

12. Alterations in Cognitive Vigilance: Kidney Failure Can Impact Cognitive Function, Resulting In Challenges With Concentration And Memory.

These Symptoms May Suggest Several Kidney Disorders Such As Chronic Kidney Disease (Ckd), Kidney Stones, Urinary Tract Infections, Or Acute

Kidney Injury. If You See Any Of These Signs Or Symptoms, It Is Important To Get Advice From A Healthcare Professional For A Thorough Evaluation And Diagnosis. Timely Identification And Action Can Effectively Control Renal Issues And Prevent Additional Complications.

CHAPTER TWO
Kidney Repair Diet Strategy

Although There Is No Miraculous "Kidney Repair Diet" To Cure Damaged Kidneys, Various Dietary Strategies Can Aid In Maintaining Kidney Health And Potentially Decelerate The Advancement Of Renal Disorders. Prior To Making Substantial Dietary Modifications, It Is Crucial To Get Guidance From A Healthcare Practitioner Or A Qualified Dietitian, Particularly For Those With Preexisting Kidney Conditions. Here Are Some Fundamental Guidelines For A Diet That Is Beneficial For Kidney Health:

1. Regulate Sodium Consumption:

• Restricting Sodium Intake Can Aid In Controlling Blood Pressure And Decreasing Fluid Accumulation. This Is Essential For Persons With Renal Issues.

2. Regulate Protein Consumption.

• It Is Crucial To Regulate Protein Consumption, Particularly For Individuals With Kidney Disease. Protein Requirements Vary Depending On An Individual's Health And Renal Function.

3. Monitor Levels Of Phosphorus And Potassium:

• Monitoring Phosphorus And Potassium Levels Is Crucial In

Advanced Renal Disease. Restrict Foods That Are Rich In These Minerals.

4. Keep Yourself Well-Hydrated:

• Proper Hydration Is Crucial For Kidney Health. Water Aids In Eliminating Waste Products And Poisons From The Body.

5. Select Nutritious Fats: Choose Sources Of Healthful Fats Including Olive Oil, Avocados, And Fatty Fish. Refrain From Consuming High Amounts Of Saturated And Trans Fats.

6. Restrict The Intake Of Added Sugars: Reducing The Intake Of Foods And Beverages High In Added Sugars

Can Aid In Weight And Blood Sugar Control, Promoting Overall Health.

7. Monitor Consumption of Foods High In Phosphorus: Some Renal Disorders May Require Limiting Foods Rich In Phosphorus, Like Dairy Products And Some Meats.

8. Moderate Intake of Coffee and Tea: While Moderate Coffee And Tea Use Is Usually Healthy, High Caffeine Intake May Need To Be Regulated For Certain Individuals.

9. Refrain From Using Alcohol: Excessive Alcohol Intake Can Lead To Dehydration And Negatively Impact Renal Function.

10.   Examine   Potassium Consumption: Individuals With Renal Issues May Need To Regulate Their Potassium Consumption, As Elevated Levels Can Be Detrimental. This Entails Restricting Specific Fruits, Vegetables, And Foods High In Potassium.

Dietary Guidelines Can Differ Depending On Individual Health Conditions And The Stage Of Renal Disease. Hence, A Customized Strategy Is Essential, And Individuals Should Collaborate Closely With Healthcare Specialists, Such As Dietitians, To Develop A Plan Suited To Their Particular Requirements.

The Efficacy Of Dietary Interventions May Vary Based On The Root Cause And Seriousness Of Renal Problems. Medical Supervision And Monitoring Are Crucial Aspects Of Renal Treatment, And Lifestyle Adjustments Should Be Done In Cooperation With Healthcare Professionals.

Essential Nutrients for Renal Health

Optimal Kidney Health Necessitates A Diet That Is Balanced And Rich In Nutrients. Various Essential Nutrients Are Vital For Maintaining Renal Function And General Health. **Below Are Essential Nutrients For Maintaining Kidney Health:**

1. Water: Proper Hydration Is Crucial For Kidney Function. Water Aids In The Elimination Of Waste Products And Pollutants, Which Helps Avoid The Development Of Kidney Stones And Promotes Overall Kidney Health.

2. Protein; Excessive Protein Consumption Can Stress The Kidneys, Thus It Is Crucial To Consume An

Appropriate Quantity Without Going Overboard. Opt For High-Quality Protein Sources Such Lean Meats, Fish, Eggs, And Plant-Based Proteins Such As Lentils.

3. Potassium: Potassium Is Crucial For Regulating Fluid Balance, Neuron Function, And Muscle Contractions. Individuals With Advanced Renal Disease May Require Monitoring And Restricting Potassium Intake. Excellent Sources Include Bananas, Oranges, Potatoes, And Leafy Green Vegetables.

4. Calcium: A Sufficient Amount Of Calcium Is Crucial For Bone Health And Has A Role In Regulating Blood Pressure. Dairy Products, Fortified

Plant-Based Milk, And Leafy Green Vegetables Are Rich In Calcium.

5. Phosphorus: Phosphorus Intake May Need To Be Controlled In Advanced Stages Of Renal Disease. Phosphorus-Rich Foods Include Dairy Products, Nuts, Seeds, And Specific Meats.

6. Vitamin D: Vitamin D Is Crucial For The Absorption Of Calcium And The Maintenance Of Bone Health. Individuals With Renal Issues May Struggle To Convert Vitamin D Into Its Active State. Sources Of Vitamin D Include Fatty Fish, Egg Yolks, And Fortified Dairy Or Plant-Based Milk.

7. Omega-3 Fatty Acids: Omega-3 Fatty Acids Include Anti-Inflammatory Characteristics And Could Potentially Improve Kidney Health. Sources Consist Of Fatty Fish Like Salmon And Mackerel, Chia Seeds, Flaxseeds, And Walnuts.

8. Antioxidants: Antioxidants Aid In Shielding The Kidneys From Oxidative Damage. Fruits And Vegetables With Vibrant Colors Like Berries, Bell Peppers, And Leafy Greens Contain High Levels Of Antioxidants.

9. Fiber: A High-Fiber Diet Promotes General Health And Can Aid In Controlling Illnesses Such As Diabetes And Obesity, Which Are Linked To Kidney Issues. Whole Grains, Fruits,

Vegetables, And Legumes Are Excellent Sources Of Dietary Fiber.

10. Vitamin B: Vitamins B Such As B6, B12, And Folic Acid Are Involved In Energy Metabolism And The Production Of Red Blood Cells. They Can Be Found In A Diverse Range Of Foods Such As Meat, Fish, Poultry, Dairy Products, And Leafy Green Vegetables.

Individual Nutrient Requirements Can Vary Depending On Factors Such As Age, Gender, Health Status, And The Existence Of Specific Medical Disorders. Individuals With Advanced Kidney Illness Should Seek Tailored Dietary Advice From Healthcare Practitioners Or Registered Dietitians

Specializing In Renal Nutrition. Consistent Monitoring And Working Closely With Healthcare Professionals Are Essential For Effectively Maintaining Kidney Health With Dietary Choices.

CHAPTER THREE
Recommended Foods for Your Diet

Following A Kidney-Friendly Diet Means Selecting Foods That Promote Kidney Health And Regulating The Consumption Of Nutrients That Could Be Detrimental In Large Quantities. Here Are Some Foods Known To Be Healthy For Kidney Health:

1. **Berries:** Berries Including Blueberries, Strawberries, And Raspberries Are Abundant In Antioxidants That Can Shield The Kidneys From Oxidative Stress.

2. **Red Capsicum:** Red Bell Peppers Have Low Potassium Levels And Are Rich In Vitamins A, C, And B6, Making

Them A Healthy Option For Kidney Health.

3. Cabbage: Cabbage Is A Suitable Vegetable For A Diet That Is Beneficial For The Kidneys Due To Its Low Levels Of Potassium And Phosphorus.

4. Cauliflower: Cauliflower Is A Flexible Vegetable With Low Potassium Levels, Making It A Suitable Alternative To High-Potassium Dishes.

5. Apples: Apples Are Rich In Fiber And Vitamin C, And Have Low Potassium Levels, Making Them Suitable For Individuals With Kidney Issues.

6. Fish: Fatty Fish Such As Salmon, Mackerel, And Trout Provide Omega-3 Fatty Acids That Possess Anti-Inflammatory Effects And Can Promote Kidney Function.

7. Olive Oil: Olive Oil Is A Heart-Healthy Fat That Can Be Used In Cooking And Salad Dressings As A Substitute For Saturated And Trans Fats.

8. Garlic: Garlic Possesses Anti-Inflammatory And Antioxidant Qualities, Making It A Tasty Addition To Meals Without The Need For Excessive Sodium.

9. Albumen: Egg Whites Are A Protein Choice That Is Excellent In Quality And Low In Phosphorus. Individuals With Renal Illness Should Regulate Their Protein Consumption According To Their Unique Requirements.

10. Cranberries: Cranberries And Cranberry Juice Can Aid In Preventing Urinary Tract Infections And Are Beneficial For Kidney Function.

11. Pineapple: Pineapple Is A Fruit With Low Potassium Levels That Offers Vitamins And Minerals, Such As Vitamin C.

12. Oats: Oats Are A Beneficial Source Of Soluble Fiber And Can Be A

Nutritious Supplement To A Diet Suitable For Renal Health.

13. White Bread and Pasta: Choose White Bread And Spaghetti Over Whole Grain Options To Lower Phosphorus Consumption.

14. Herbs and Spices: Use Herbs And Spices Such As Basil, Parsley, Thyme, And Lemon Zest To Enhance The Flavor Of Foods Without Using Salt.

15. Water: Maintaining Proper Hydration Is Essential For Kidney Health. Water Aids In The Removal Of Waste Products And Poisons From The Body.

Individual Dietary Requirements Can Differ Depending On Things Like Renal

Function, Overall Health, And Specific Medical Problems. Seeking Guidance From A Healthcare Practitioner Or A Registered Dietitian Specializing In Renal Nutrition Helps Customize Dietary Advice To Meet Individual Needs And Promote Optimal Kidney Health.

Limit or Avoid These Foods

People With Renal Disorders Or Individuals Seeking To Enhance Kidney Function Should Be Cautious Of Some Meals That Could Exacerbate Kidney Problems. **Here Are Foods To Restrict Or Exclude In A Kidney-Friendly Diet:**

1. Foods High In Sodium: Limit Processed Foods, Canned Soups, Deli Meats, And Salty Snacks To Reduce Sodium Intake, Which Can Lead To Elevated Blood Pressure And Fluid Retention.

2. Convenience and Quick-Service Foods: Fast Food And Processed Meals Typically Have Elevated Levels Of Sodium, Harmful Fats, And Additives That Can Have Adverse Effects On Kidney Function.

3. Foods Rich in Potassium: Some Fruits And Vegetables Like Bananas, Oranges, Tomatoes, And Potatoes Are Rich In Potassium. Individuals With Kidney Issues May Need To Restrict Their Consumption And Keep An Eye

On Their Potassium Levels, Even Though These Foods Can Be Included In A Well-Rounded Diet.

4. Foods High In Phosphorus: Phosphorus-Rich Foods Like Dairy Products, Nuts, Seeds, And Certain Meats May Require Restriction, Particularly In Advanced Kidney Disease.

5. Colas with a Dark Hue: Colas And Other Dark Sodas Contain Phosphoric Acid, Which Can Increase The Risk Of Kidney Stone Formation.

6. Protein-Rich Foods: Protein Is Necessary, But Consuming Too Much Can Put A Strain On The Kidneys. People With Kidney Issues Should

Regulate Their Protein Consumption And Prioritize High-Quality Protein Sources.

7. Charcuterie: Processed Meats Such As Bacon, Sausages, And Hot Dogs Are Rich In Sodium And May Contain Additives That Could Be Detrimental To Kidney Function.

8. Avoiding Foods High In Oxalate: Individuals At Risk Of Kidney Stones Should Consider Restricting Foods Rich In Oxalates, Like Beets, Chocolate, And Nuts.

9. Restricting Phosphate Additives: Processed Foods Frequently Include Phosphate Additives, Which May Lead To Elevated Phosphorus Levels. It Is

Crucial To Read Food Labels And Opt For Low-Phosphorus Alternatives.

10. Foods High In Oxalate: Some People May Have To Restrict High-Oxalate Foods Like Spinach, Rhubarb, And Beet Greens To Lower The Chances Of Developing Kidney Stones.

11. Alcohol: Excessive Alcohol Intake Can Lead To Dehydration And Negatively Impact Renal Function. Avoid Excessive Alcohol Consumption And Ensure Proper Hydration.

12. Caffeine: Excessive Caffeine Consumption Can Lead To Dehydration, Although Moderate Intake Is Usually Safe. Those With

Renal Problems Should Regulate Their Consumption Of Caffeine.

It Is Essential For Individuals With Kidney Issues To Collaborate Closely With Healthcare Professionals, Such As Dietitians, To Customize Dietary Advice According To Their Unique Requirements. Consistent Monitoring And Dietary Adjustments According To Kidney Function And Overall Health Are Crucial For Preserving Kidney Health And Avoiding Additional Complications.

CHAPTER FOUR
Meal Planning and Recipes

To Plan Meals For Kidney Health, Choose Foods That Are Rich In Nutrients And Carefully Monitor The Consumption Of Sodium, Potassium, Phosphorus, And Protein. **Here Is A Sample Meal Plan Along With Kidney-Friendly Meals To Inspire You.**

Exemplary Meal Plan:

Breakfast: Scrambled Egg Whites with Spinach and Red Bell Peppers

• Whole Grain Toast (Reduce Intake If Monitoring Phosphorus Levels)

• Fresh Berries

Lunch: Grilled Chicken Salad with Mixed Greens, Cucumber, and Cherry Tomatoes

• Dressing Made With Olive Oil and Lemon

• Quinoa (Restrict If Monitoring Phosphorus Levels)

Snack: Greek Yogurt Parfait with Low-Potassium Fruits Such As Berries and a Sprinkle of Granola

Dinner: Baked Salmon With Lemon And Herbs.

• Steamed Asparagus (Reduce Intake If Monitoring Phosphorus Levels)

• Cauliflower Puree (As a Replacement for Mashed Potatoes)

Snack: Fresh Fruit Salad with Low-Potassium Options Such As Apples and Grapes.

Recipes Suitable For Individuals with Kidney Conditions:

1. Grilled Chicken and Vegetable Skewers:

Ingredients: Chicken Breast, Bell Peppers, Cherry Tomatoes, Olive Oil, Garlic, Herbs.

Marinate The Chicken In A Mixture Of Olive Oil, Garlic, And Herbs. Thread Chicken and Vegetables onto Skewers and Heat Until Done.

2. Quinoa and Vegetable Stir-Fry:

Ingredients: Quinoa, Broccoli, Carrots, Snap Peas, Low-Sodium Soy Sauce, Ginger, Garlic.

Cook Quinoa and Sauté Vegetables with Ginger and Garlic. Combine Cooked Quinoa With Soy Sauce.

3. Baked Salmon with Lemon and Dill:

Ingredients: Salmon Fillets, Lemon, Fresh Dill, Olive Oil, Garlic.

Season The Salmon With Olive Oil, Lemon, Dill, And Garlic. Cook Until The Salmon Easily Breaks Into Flakes.

4. Mashed Cauliflower:

Ingredients: Cauliflower, Low-Fat Milk, Garlic, Salt, Pepper.

Steam Cauliflower, Then Puree With Low-Fat Milk, Garlic, Salt, And Pepper Until A Smooth Consistency Is Achieved.

5. Berry and Yogurt Parfait:

Ingredients: Greek Yogurt, Low-Potassium Berries Such As Blueberries and Strawberries, Granola.

There Is No Text Provided.Create A Delicious Parfait By Layering Greek Yogurt With Berries And Oats.

6. Fresh Fruit Salad:

Ingredients: Apples, Grapes, Kiwi, Mint Leaves.

Combine Diced Fruits, Sprinkle With Lemon Juice, and Decorate With Mint Leaves.

Be Sure To Modify Serving Amounts and Particular Ingredients According To Individual Dietary Requirements And Limitations. It Is Recommended To Get Guidance From A Healthcare Practitioner Or A Qualified Dietitian To Develop A Customized Meal Plan Tailored To Your Individual Kidney Health Needs.

Physical Activity and Renal Health

Consistent Physical Activity Is Essential For Preserving General Well-Being, Which Includes Aiding Kidney Function. Here Are Several Ways Exercise Improves Kidney Health:

• Physical Activity Assists in Regulating Blood Pressure, Hence Decreasing the Likelihood Of Hypertension. Hypertension Is A Primary Contributor To Kidney Injury.

• **Enhanced Cardiovascular Health:** Exercise Leads To Improved Cardiovascular Health, Therefore Benefiting Renal Function. An Efficient Cardiovascular System Guarantees

Enough Blood Circulation To The Kidneys.

• **Weight Management:** Maintaining A Healthy Weight Through Consistent Physical Activity Might Lower The Likelihood Of Acquiring Illnesses Such As Diabetes And Obesity, Which Are Linked To Kidney Issues.

• Exercise Helps Regulate Blood Sugar Levels, Decreasing The Likelihood Of Developing Diabetes. Diabetes Is A Major Contributor To The Development Of Renal Disease.

• Enhanced Insulin Sensitivity Due To Frequent Physical Activity Reduces Load On The Kidneys Caused By Insulin Resistance.

• Chronic Inflammation Is Associated With Renal Damage. Consistent Physical Activity Reduces Inflammation In The Body.

• Exercise Helps Prevent Kidney Stone Formation By Improving Adequate Hydration And Reducing Risk Factors Linked To Stone Formation.

• Regular Strength Training Exercises Aid in Preserving Muscular Mass, Which Is Crucial For Overall Health, Including Renal Function.

• **Enhanced Mood And Mental Health:** Physical Activity Is Recognized For Its Ability To Boost Mood And Mental Well-Being. Stress And Mental Health Problems Can

Affect General Health, Including Kidney Function.

• Regular Exercise Boosts Immunological Function, Decreasing The Likelihood Of Illnesses That May Impact The Kidneys.

Exercise Recommendations:

• Participate In Cardiovascular Exercises Like Walking, Running, Cycling, Swimming, Or Dancing For A Minimum Of 150 Minutes Each Week, As Advised By Health Recommendations.

• Engage In Strength Training Exercises At Least Twice A Week To Preserve Muscular Mass. Concentrate

On Primary Muscular Groups With Correct Technique.

• Flexibility And Stretching: O Incorporate Flexibility Exercises To Increase Joint Range Of Motion And Lower The Chance Of Injury.

• Maintain Proper Water Levels, Particularly Before And After Physical Activity, To Promote Kidney Function And Avoid Dehydration.

• Utilize An Individualized Approach By Seeking Guidance From Healthcare Professionals Such As Doctors Or Fitness Experts To Create A Personalized Workout Regimen Based On Your Specific Health Condition And Medical History.

Prior To Commencing A New Fitness Regimen, Particularly For Persons With Preexisting Health Concerns, It Is Crucial To Seek Guidance From A Healthcare Practitioner To Confirm That The Selected Activities Are Safe And Suitable For Individual Requirements.

CHAPTER FIVE
Diet Suitable For Individuals with Diabetes and Kidney Issues

Individuals With Diabetes And Renal Issues Should Adhere To A Kidney-Friendly Diet That Aids In Controlling Blood Sugar Levels. Here Are Dietary Recommendations To Follow For A Kidney-Friendly Diet Tailored For Those With Diabetes:

1. Regulate Portion Sizes:

• Monitoring Portion Sizes Is Essential For Controlling Calorie Consumption, Which Is Important For Managing Weight And Regulating Blood Sugar Levels.

2. Select Lean Protein Sources To Effectively Manage Diabetes And Renal

Health. Examples Consist Of Skinless Fowl, Fish, Eggs, Tofu, And Beans.

3. Restrict Phosphorus and Potassium:

• People With Kidney Problems Should Regulate Their Phosphorus And Potassium Consumption. Select Foods That Are Low In Phosphorus And Potassium. This May Require Restricting Specific Fruits, Vegetables, And Dairy Items.

4. Monitor Sodium Intake:

Restricting Sodium Intake Aids In Controlling Blood Pressure And Decreasing Fluid Retention. Select Fresh, Unprocessed Meals And Utilize

Herbs And Spices For Taste Rather Than Salt.

5. Prioritize Whole Grains:

• Opt For Whole Grains Such As Brown Rice, Quinoa, And Whole Wheat Over Refined Grains. Whole Grains Offer Fiber, Which Is Advantageous For Diabetes And Kidney Health.

6. Incorporate Nutritious Fats Like Olive Oil, Avocados, And Fatty Seafood, Which Are Beneficial For Heart Health. These Fats Can Aid In Regulating Cholesterol Levels.

7. Maintain Proper Fluids To Support Kidney Health. Supervise Fluid Consumption, Particularly If Limited By Kidney Problems.

8. Monitor Blood Glucose Levels Regularly And Collaborate With Healthcare Providers To Modify The Diet As Needed. Take Into Account The Glycemic Index Of Foods To Assist In Controlling Blood Sugar Fluctuations.

Meal Suggestions:

Breakfast: Oatmeal Topped With Fresh Berries And Chia Seeds.

• Scrambled Eggs with Spinach and Tomatoes.

Lunch: Grilled Chicken Salad With Mixed Greens, Cucumbers, And Light Vinaigrette.

• Stir-Fried Quinoa and Vegetables with Tofu.

Snack Options:

Greek Yogurt with Almonds

Sliced Apples With Peanut Butter.

Dinner: Baked Fish Seasoned With Lemon And Dill.

• Brown Rice or Cauliflower Rice.

• Asparagus Steamed.

Snack: Carrot Sticks With Hummus.

• Berries Topped With Whipped Cream, If Dietary Restrictions Allow.

Key Factors:

• Always Get Advice From A Certified Dietician Or Healthcare Expert To Develop A Customized Meal Plan Tailored To Unique Health Needs.

• Frequently Check Blood Glucose Levels and Modify the Diet Accordingly.

• Adhere To Medication Regimen And Medical Guidance To Effectively Control Diabetes And Maintain Renal Health.

Customized Nutrition Programs Are Crucial Due To The Variability Of Dietary Requirements Influenced By The Extent Of Kidney Disease, Medications, And Other Health Considerations. Consistent Check-Ins With Healthcare Professionals Help Maintain The Suitability And Efficacy Of The Eating Plan.

Pharmaceuticals And Nutritional Supplements

Supplements And Drugs Are Essential For Maintaining Kidney Health, Particularly For Persons With Renal Disease Or Related Diseases. It Is Crucial To Consider That Tailored Suggestions May Differ Depending On One's Health Condition, The Progression Of Renal Disease, And Additional Variables. Always Consult With Healthcare Specialists Before Starting Any New Supplements Or Medications. Here Are Some Prevalent Factors To Consider:

Supplements:

1. Individuals With Renal Disease May Struggle To Convert Vitamin D Into Its Active Form. Supplementing With Vitamin D May Be Advised To Promote Bone Health. Dosage Should Be Determined According To The Results Of Blood Tests.

2. Iron Deficiency Is A Prevalent Consequence Of Renal Illness. Iron Supplements Might Be Administered To Treat Low Hemoglobin Levels.

3. Calcium Supplements May Be Advised To Promote Bone Health Based On Dietary Limitations And Laboratory Findings. It Is Crucial To Maintain A Balance Between Calcium

Consumption And Other Minerals Such As Phosphorus.

4. Omega-3 Fatty Acids, Including Those Found In Fish Oil Capsules, May Provide Anti-Inflammatory Advantages. Seek Advice From Healthcare Professionals To Establish Suitable Dosages.

5. Individuals With Renal Illness May Need B Vitamin Supplements Like B12 And Folic Acid To Treat Deficiencies And Promote General Health.

6. Phosphate Binders Are Prescribed In Severe Renal Disease To Regulate Phosphorus Levels In The Blood.

7. Erythropoiesis-Stimulating Agents (Esas) Such Erythropoietin Can Be

Used To Boost Red Blood Cell Synthesis In People With Anemia Linked To Kidney Disease.

Prescribed Drugs:

1. Ace Inhibitors Or Arbs Are Frequently Administered To Treat Hypertension And Safeguard The Kidneys.

2. Diuretics Are Recommended To Treat Fluid Retention, A Frequent Consequence Of Renal Illness.

3. Statins Are Used To Regulate Cholesterol Levels And Lower The Chances Of Cardiovascular Issues.

4. Phosphate Binders Are Recommended To Regulate Phosphorus Levels In The Blood.

5. Potassium Binders Are Prescribed In Cases Of Hyperkalemia To Eliminate Excess Potassium From The Body.

6. Nonsteroidal Anti-Inflammatory Medicines (NSAIDS) Should Be Avoided Due To Their Potential To Cause Kidney Damage. Alternative Methods For Managing Pain May Be Suggested.

Factors to Take Into Account:

• **Regular Monitoring:** O It Is Crucial To Do Routine Blood Tests And Check-Ups To Oversee Kidney Function, Modify Medications, And Manage Any Possible Consequences.

• **Personalized Treatment:** Treatment Programs Are Tailored To

Each Individual. Healthcare Practitioners Take Into Account The Individual Demands, Renal Function, And Other Medical Issues Of The Patient.

- **Compliance:** It Is Essential To Follow The Prescribed Drugs And Supplements For Optimal Management. Adhere To Medication Instructions Provided By Healthcare Professionals.

It Is Essential To Freely Speak With Healthcare Specialists On Any Concerns, Side Effects, Or Changes In Health Status. They Offer Tailored Advice Considering The Person's General Well-Being And Particular Renal Ailment.

Conclusion

Ultimately, It Is Crucial To Prioritize Kidney Health For General Wellness, And Taking A Proactive And Knowledgeable Stance Can Aid In The Prevention And Treatment Of Kidney-Related Problems. Key Aspects To Concentrate On Are:

• Adhere To A Kidney-Friendly Diet That Maintains A Balance Of Important Nutrients While Regulating Salt, Potassium, Phosphorus, And Protein Consumption. Include Fresh Fruits, Veggies, Lean Proteins, And Whole Grains.

• Hydration Is Crucial For Kidney Function And Overall Health. Drink Enough Water To Stay Well-Hydrated.

• Engage In Consistent Physical Exercise To Promote Cardiovascular Health, Regulate Blood Pressure, Manage Blood Sugar Levels, And Sustain A Healthy Weight.

• **Monitoring And Testing:** Regularly Check Blood Pressure, Blood Sugar Levels, And Kidney Function Using Suitable Tests. Timely Intervention Is Possible With Early Detection.

• Follow Healthcare Professionals' Instructions For Taking Prescribed Drugs And Supplements. Address Any Worries Or Possible Adverse Reactions With Your Healthcare Professionals.

- Consult Healthcare Professionals Such As Nephrologists, Dietitians, And Primary Care Physicians Often To Develop Personalized Programs For Kidney Health.

- **Lifestyle Choices:** - Adopt Lifestyle Habits That Promote Kidney Health By Refraining From Smoking, Reducing Alcohol Use, And Utilizing Healthy Stress Management Techniques.

- **Individualized Approach:** - Acknowledge That Every Person Has Unique Health Requirements. Collaborate With Healthcare Specialists To Customize Advice For Specific Illnesses Like Diabetes Or Other Underlying Health Concerns.

- **Education And Awareness:** - Keep Yourself Updated On Kidney Health And The Risk Factors Linked To Renal Disease. Education Enables Individuals To Make Knowledgeable Choices Regarding Their Health.

- **Early Intervention:** Promptly Seek Medical Assistance If You Observe Any Indications Or Symptoms Of Kidney Issues. Timely Intervention Can Greatly Influence Results And Halt The Advancement Of Renal Disease.

Keep In Mind That Kidney Health Is Essential For General Well-Being, And A Comprehensive Strategy That Includes Lifestyle, Diet, And Medical Care Is Vital For Preserving Normal Kidney Function. Always Seek Advice

From Healthcare Specialists For Tailored Recommendations And Prompt Intervention.

THE END